The Head, Neck & Shoulder Pain Bible: A Self-Care Guide To Eliminating Upper Body Pain

****

Copyright © 2018 Christopher J. Kidawski
ISBN: 9781724397966

****

Published by Influential Health Solutions LLC in Lighthouse Point, Fl. All Rights Reserved Worldwide. No part of this book may be reproduced in any way without written consent from the author.

DISCLAIMER:

No part of this publication may be reproduced or transmitted in any form or by any means, mechanical or electronic, including photocopying or recording, or by any information storage and retrieval system, or transmitted by email without permission in writing from the author.

Neither the author nor the publisher assumes any responsibility for errors, omissions, or contrary interpretations of the subject matter herein. Any perceived slight of any individual or organization is purely unintentional.

Brand and product names are trademarks or registered trademarks of their respective owners.

Although the exercises depicted in this book are restorative, nothing contained in this book is meant to treat, or cure any diseases. The use of any object to release muscle tissue can be dangerous by pressing on internal organs and unseen nerves. Practicing anything in this book by you, the reader, completely absolves the author of any wrongdoing as you are doing so at your own risk. As with any type of exercises program, please consult your physician before you start.

Also By Chris

The Death Of Dieting: Lose Weight, Banish Allergies, and Feed Your Body What It Needs To Thrive!

The Everspace: Utilizing the Power Of God and Neuroscience To Create Stillness Within.

The Back Pain Bible: A Breakthrough Step-By-Step Self-Treatment Process To End Chronic Pain Forever!

The Knee Pain Bible: A Self-Care Guide to Eliminating Knee Pain and Returning to The Movements You Love!

The Foot & Ankle Pain Bible: A Self-Care Guide to Eliminating The Source of Your Foot Pain.

Not Your Average Paleo Diet Cookbook: 100 Delicious & Healthy (Mostly) Lectin-Free Recipes!

Not Your Average Vegan Instant Pot Cookbook: 100 Delicious & Healthy Recipes!

Not Your Average Paleo Cookbook: 100 Delicious & Healthy (Mostly) Lectin-Free Recipes!

The Head, Neck & Shoulder Pain Bible
A Self-Care Guide to Eliminating Upper Body Pain

Christopher J. Kidawski

Dedication

For Andrea, and a lifetime of fixing you…

Foreword

Progress is what humans make. No one can deny that everything we do in life is for the pursuit of progress. Even if we are not actively pursuing progress, it manifests itself in one way or another in our minds and bodies. We pursue it in our jobs, with our families, in our financial endeavors, our personal development, in training, in learning, and in becoming.

There is always the next step, the next stop, the next waypoint, obstacle, finish line, and the next starting line. Progress can be negative, positive, neutral, made, lost, gained, given, and taken. Every person will experience each of these modes of progress in life no matter the road that they travel, and each form holds a map to the next measure of progress to be encountered.

Enough philosophy. If you are physically active, you are going to get hurt or injured. Accept this and continue to make progress by means that are practiced and proven. Not everything needs surgery. In fact, my personal belief is that you should exhaust every other means of correction prior to going under the knife. With the increasing popularity of recreational fitness, and the increase in occupations that require you remain physically capable, surgery can be a form of negative progress. Regrettably, it is often unnecessary as well. This isn't to say that surgery isn't sometimes needed. But if you are experiencing discomfort, loss of ability, loss of mobility and or pain, try the methods in this book first.

    My job requires that I remain physically able and physically competitive. I view it as a part of my occupation that each day I exercise, build my strength, increase my endurance, hone my speed and form and perform routine maintenance on my body and its abilities. And of course I am still a human, so I get hurt.

    This was the case with my shoulder, or so I thought. I don't know where this most recent injury came form. It just started hurting one day. This was problematic because I couldn't tell anyone how I hurt it. No one could examine my movements to come up with a probable cause. It just hurt. I trained through it for a couple of weeks, and it continued to get worse. My problem was that I could not describe exactly what the pain was or where it came from. Luckily, I knew a guy, and after swallowing much pride, I approached CK and asked him to have a look at my issues. CK did his work and I was honest with him. There was an instance where I got up from doing the exercises and he gave me the routine "how does it feel?" To which I replied, "nothing has changed." Later that night I received a battery of text messages and screenshots with drawings of my problem area with certain areas highlighted and circled and noted, all from CK interrogating me about my pain. Totally unexpected. I thought that he would just accept my word for words and move on to the next client. The man took the time at his house and studied my problem! After we reached a verdict, the next treatment was immensely effective. And the treatment after that, more so. And the treatment after that, even more so.

This rounds out two points that I want to give you about the literature in your hands. The author knows about your problem and is willing to find it and fix it, but it also takes time and determination to get better. Repeat after me, *it takes time.* Do not become frustrated if you follow the instructions and guidance in this book and it is not better after the first, second, or third session. Remember, you are seeking progress. You don't lose the weight in a day. You don't beat every personal record in a day. And you don't see or feel the results from a massage in a day. Be patient and make progress. That's what I did, and it worked for the extreme measures I put myself through.

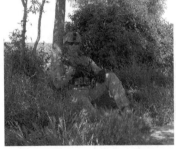

Aaron G.
Captain USMC

Table of Contents

Dedication

Foreword

Introduction: Pain = Confusion, Confusion = More Pain

    Chapter 1: The Atlas - When Your Foundation Gets Funky
    The Bone
    The Muscles
    Fixing The Problem
    The Mysteriously Elevated Shoulder
    Last, But Not Least

Ask The Coach: Are You a Chiro Hater, Or What?

    Chapter 2: Birds of a Feather Flock Together – Head & Neck Pain
    Your Angry Muscle Tissue
    Masters of Chaos – The Scalenes
    The Sternocleidomastoid (SCM)
    The Trapezius
    The Levator Scapulae
    The Rhomboids
    The Splenius Muscles

Ask the Coach: Do You Recommend a Specific Pillow?

    Chapter 3: Where Your Shoulder Pain Is Really Coming From

It's Not Me, It's You
Front of the Shoulder Pain
  The Infraspinatus
  The Supraspinatus
  The Teres Minor
  The Subscapularis
  The Scalenes
  The Subclavius
  Pec Major & Minor
  The Biceps
Back of the Shoulder Pain
  The Teres Major
  The Serratus Posterior Superior
  The Latissimus Dorsi
  The Triceps

Ask the Coach: What About Stretching the Shoulder?
  Chapter 4: Special Considerations
  Motion Sickness
  Vertigo
  TMJ

Concluding Thoughts
About The Author

Introduction: Pain = Confusion, Confusion = More Pain

With all of the books on the market that deal with head, neck, and shoulder pain I'm sure you're wondering right now how this one sets itself apart and could possibly help you. While stating facts in my profession is a bold move, I can say this with the utmost certainty – any pain you have had in your upper body, I've probably had at one point or another in my life as well. And if I haven't had the same pain as you, I'm 100 percent certain I have helped someone get rid of the same pain you're experiencing.

Among all the other ailments I've written about in my books, head, neck, and shoulder pain are the most prevalent for people – even beating out back pain in my opinion. The reason why back pain gets so much attention is because of how vicious it can be when we have it. Case in point, the number-one reason people call into sick for work is because of back pain, while the number-one excuse people give to get out of being intimate with their partner is a headache, which is hardly noteworthy.

In all honesty, I'm not trying to downplay your pain or diminish it. I have had several people come to me physically crying, telling me about their neck pain, shoulder pain, vertigo, TMJ, or migraines. They all say the same thing. They all have been to the best doctors, chiropractors, and physical therapists. None have found an ounce of relief. Their pain used to just affect the way they exercised, or whether they would stay out late at a party or not. Now it is all consuming.

The reason why head, neck, and shoulder pain is so hard to treat is because the closer pain is to the brain, the harder it is for your brain to pinpoint where it is coming from. Couple that with the fact that your brain can only register your top three pains in the body at any moment, and the fact that trigger points can refer pain into parts of the body where a problem is not present, and you have a trifecta of tail-chasing going on. The solutions in this book are going to help you stop chasing your tail (pain), and help you figure out what's really going on (where's your problem).

As you'll see from the very first chapter, most practitioners have pain remediation completely wrong. The era my father grew up in during the 50s and 60s heralded the doctor as the end all be all king of medicine. It didn't matter if his or her methods were outdated – you took a doctor's word for gospel truth. Nowadays people are questioning more and getting harder to fool. If my neck pain hasn't improved after three chiropractic adjustments, why will 15 more make it better? If my shoulder isn't better after three months of physical therapy, why will six months make a difference? If my migraines are getting worse even with medication, then what is the medication really doing for me? These are all questions we are going to explore and answer in hopes of making you what I call, "Your own best therapist."

Now I'm not trying to talk down on doctors (two of my cousins are doctors), therapists, or chiropractors. What I'm trying to say is that our understanding of the human body has taken a drastic turn for the better in the last few years. For instance, Jean-Claude Guimberteau published a book called, *The Architechture of Human Living Fascia* in October of 2015. He was sitting on nearly 20 years of secrets about how the body really works and finally decided to let the cat out of the bag.

What Guimberteau discovered was that living fascia was quite different than the dead fascia we studied in cadavers. Living fascia is a covering of collagen and water filled tubes that sits between the skin and the muscle tissue. It penetrates everything and in doing so connects everything in the body. The therapists in my circle say, "What happens in the toes can be felt in the nose." Really understanding and believing in this view of how the body works when it comes to pain will help make sense of what you are going to read in the rest of this book.

Guimberteau's discoveries on fascia have confirmed what I have been figuring out and dealing with for the last 12 years. Questions like, "Why does it hurt in your arm, when I press in your shoulder?" Or, "Why is your left shoulder hurting, when we press into your right?" Guimberteau brought all of this to light by scientifically showing us that fascia is not only a living component to our body (we thought it was inert), but that it is actually the master control center for the entire human body, especially when it comes to movement and pain. Honing in on pain and then launching a scud missile at it in the form of injections or surgery is like killing a single ant with a stick of dynamite and expecting the colony to die. The body just doesn't work as simply as we thought it did.

In my opinion, because of these new findings, most doctors are just not qualified to deal with pain anymore. Pills and shots for joint pain will only produce more people who used to be productive members of society but are now hooked on opioids. Chiropractors, physical therapists, and anyone who is "specializing" in one specific area of the body are only treating your symptoms, rather than fixing your problem. I don't care if you have four herniated disks in your neck or you just stubbed your toe, your injury needs to be looked at from a total body perspective; not from an isolationist point of view.

Let me once again ease the critics shaking their heads right now. I'm not saying these professions are worthless or they should all be forced to shut down. All of the practitioners mentioned have helped millions of people combined I'm sure. What I'm saying is that when it comes to pain, specifically chronic pain, you need someone like me to do your dirty work for you. You need what is called a "structural" therapist.

What is structural therapy? Structural therapy is kind of like this – let's say you own the Empire State building and a 6.4 magnitude earth quake happens. People are rattled, but the building withstood the quake. You now have two options to check and see what damage was done – the janitor who has been with you for 40 years and knows every room like the back of your hand or a structural engineer. My money is on you choosing the engineer.

When I look at a human being, I see a juxtaposition of terms. We are machines, but we are also webs. The funny thing about us is you can exchange an old heart for a new one just as you can exchange a crappy carburetor in a car for a new one, but you can never remove fascia from the human body. Our fascia is with us from about two weeks after we are conceived and only leaves us when we decompose.

Modern medicine looks at the body as if we have 600 muscles, which would be true on any anatomy chart. No doctor in his or her right mind would call another doctor crazy for operating on your shoulder if you were having severe enough pain in it. The shoulder muscle must be dysfunctional and in need of repair. In my world, shoulder pain is manifested as an offset atlas bone, a tight anterior scalene muscle, a tight pec minor muscle, a tight infraspinatus muscle, a tight subscapularis muscle, or a tight latissimus dorsi – all of which can be manually loosened up to resolve the pain you are experiencing. I've seen it happen 1,000 times – literally.

I'm sure you can agree with me that the health professions would take a pretty big hit if everyone was running out to buy lacrosse balls, baseballs, and softballs to relieve their ailments. If their patients had the knowledge I did, there would be no big pharma companies knocking on their doors with a fat check for prescribing their medications. Hence, their hands are tied. But enough talk about what doesn't work. You already know all of this – maybe not as eloquently, but deep down inside you know what you have been doing has not been working or else you wouldn't have this book in your hand.

Throughout this book I am going to present real world cases of people just like you, people who came to me with the exact type of pain you have.

I'm then going to show you how to *permanently* get rid of it, just as I did in my clients. A quick note before we bang this drum – because the brain gets confused the closer pain is to it, the body becomes very good at hiding where the pain is actually coming from. When you are mobilizing an area, pay close attention to see if there is any other pain being referred and to where it is going. These are what I call hotspots (trigger points) – where your pain actually is, compared to where you feel it. You may be scratching your head a little right now, but as you will see, this will all make sense soon enough.

For more information, or to join my e-mail list, please go to www.chriskidawski.com

If you read this entire book, have applied the methods and still continue to have pain, feel free to contact me for a consultation at rebuildingu@proton.me

Follow me on Instagram: @thepainbibles

At this point, I would like to extend my truest gratitude and deepest appreciation for you supporting me and my business. Don't ever feel like you are alone in this battle to be pain free.

CK
Honolulu, Hawai'i
May 15, 2018

Chapter 1: The Atlas - When Your Foundation Gets Funky

Aaron, a highly skilled Marine, came to me with a pretty funky issue. A specimen of warfare, he stands 6'2" and weighs 225 pounds. During our consultation, he was complaining of a pain that he couldn't really put into words. It was in the left side of his neck, and travelled into his chest. He had a hard time taking a deep breath, and he would get lightheaded frequently as well. A secondary problem was his back pain. It would go out whenever it felt like it, he said, and it was very frustrating considering he ran six miles a day with a 60lb backpack on.

During our first session, I had him work extensively on his left side neck, his left shoulder, and his left chest muscle. When he returned, he said it was better, but not completely gone. This went on for two more sessions, which frustrated me to no end because if my clients are not getting better, that means I am off the mark.

Since his body was telling me to look elsewhere, that is exactly what I did. I had Aaron dig into a reflexive point in his shoulder for his Atlas bone and what ensued was pure muscle geek comedy. First the pain shot across into his left shoulder, then down into his left chest, then back up across to his right shoulder, down his right arm, and then into his right side upper back before diminishing with a slight popping feeling. How do I know all of this? Because he literally gave me a play by play as it was all going on.

Aaron was amazed, and could not believe what he had just experienced. I just smiled at the wonderment of how the body works. When Aaron returned for his last appointment, he said that the pain was down to about 5 percent and getting better every day.

This case was special to me because Aaron was set to train for seven weeks for Marine Special Operations Command (MARSOC), so I had a time crunch going on as I could not let him endure more pain than he was already experiencing. To my delight, he completed the training and was accepted into his new role in the Marines. Semper Fi! Hoo Rah!

The Bone

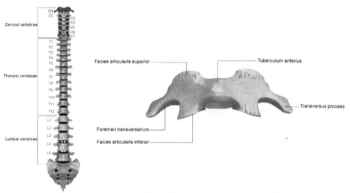

Cervical vertebrae C1: Anterior view

If you've read a copy of my book *The Foot & Ankle Pain Bible,* you might have noticed a little cliffhanger. I talk about one of my mentors, Ida Rolf, and how she coined the saying, "All problems start with the feet." While in some cases that may be true, in my opinion our true foundation is the atlas, not our feet. When you talk about what a foundation really is – being a base of support – then the foot seems to fit that fairly well. The problem to me is that the body is always going to follow the head as far as movement is concerned. If the head is off, the feet are going to be off, but the inverse is not true. Our feet can be off, but our head can be straight.

If there is one thing that I see destroying more and more people's ability to function it's an offset atlas, Your atlas is your first cervical vertebrae upon which your skull sits. The bone just below is called your axis. Tunneling down the middle of both of these vertebrae is your brainstem, which not only controls but also coordinates virtually all of your body's functions. When damage occurs to either of these two vertebrae, the connective tissue (fascia), or muscles surrounding the bones, the atlas and the axis can misalign and lock into a stressed abnormal position. As a result of the abnormal pressure, tension, and irritation, there will be a disruption of blood flow as well as cerebrospinal fluid circulating around this area. You are basically choking off the signals your brain is sending to the rest of your body from the launching point. Total body chaos ensues.

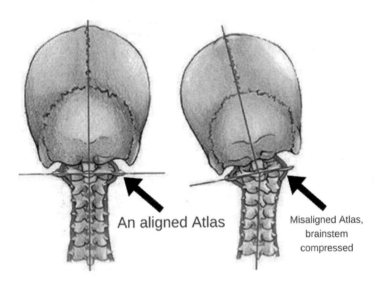

An aligned Atlas

Misaligned Atlas, brainstem compressed

The most critical aspect of this injury to note is that an Atlas subluxation will remain stuck in this abnormal position, slowly causing health problems over time with the average time to onset of symptoms being 10-15 years. Here is a laundry list of health problems this simple misalignment can create, according to the Upper Cervical Health Center:

1. Neck pain, stiffness, muscle ache.
2. Headaches that frequently involve the base of the skull and radiate usually to one side of the head.
3. Migraine's that not only produce a throbbing pain but may cause visual disturbance, nausea, or vomiting.
4. Vertigo, dizziness, faintness, ringing in the ears (tinnitus) and some types of hearing loss.
5. Facial pain or palsy.
6. Grating or crackling sounds at the base of the skull when turning your head.
7. Inability to fully turn or lean your head to one side or the other (loss of range of motion).
8. Shoulder pain that is commonly between the shoulder blades but can occur between the neck and shoulder area as well.
9. Jaw pain that is typically behind the jaw or close to the ear.
10. Postural distortion:
    a. Head tilt
    b. Shoulder tilt
    c. Pelvic tilt

    d. Short leg
    e. Head, shoulder, rib cage, and pelvic rotation can also occur.
11. Chest or rib ache, discomfort, or pain from postural distortion.
12. Nerve root irritation can occur at the resulting stress points along the spine.
13. Radiating arm pain, shoulder pain and leg pain (sciatica) can develop through nerve root tension and irritation.
14. Low back pain and spinal disc damage occur over time due to postural distortion.
15. Hip, knee, or ankle pain and dysfunction typically on the side of the short leg.
16. Brain congestion due to mechanical blockage of blood flow, particularly venous drainage and cerebrospinal fluid circulation. (Current research is pointing to neurodegenerative disorders developing over time due to long-term brain congestion).
17. High blood pressure (neurologically based).
18. Vagus nerve disruption presented as heart, lung, stomach, digestive, and bowl disorders.
19. An imbalance between sympathetic (fight or flight system) and parasympathetic (rest and digest system) nervous system, which most commonly results in over-activity of the fight or flight response leading to a chronic stress state.
20. Difficulty sleeping, insomnia and in some cases grind of their teeth at night.
21. Numbness and tingling in all extremities.
22. Inability to take a deep breath/locked up breathing.

23. Postural Orthostatic Tachycardia Syndrome (POTS)

That's a pretty long list of health problems a funky atlas can cause wouldn't you say? Symptom number 23 is actually my own addition to the list. POTS is receiving a lot of buzz in the news lately, but if you look at the symptoms of POTS and compare them to a misaligned atlas – they are nearly identical. Here are just of few examples of symptoms people with POTS experience:

- Blurred vision
- Lightheadedness, dizziness or fainting
- Heart palpitations
- Headache
- Poor concentration
- Tiredness
- Gastrointestinal symptoms (for example, nausea, cramps, bloating, constipation, diarrhea)
- Shortness of breath
- Head, neck or chest discomfort
- Weakness
- Sleep disorders
- Difficulty exercising
- Anxiety
- Coldness or pain in the extremities

When we dive deeper and look at the causes of POTS, nearly every website states that the

causes of this condition are poorly understood. Causes of POTS are listed as starting after:
1. Major surgery - being invasive sets off alarm bells in the body causing the brain to lock down muscle groups to protect joints.
2. Pregnancy – Carrying a weighted load (the baby) for 9 months plus the strain of delivery or C-Section can stress the spine including the atlas.
3. Trauma – A car accident or hard fall can jar the skull locking the atlas in a poor position.
4. Viral illness – Laying in bed for days on end in poor positions will definitely lock up the atlas. How many times have you woken up with a stiff neck?

All I see when I read that list is fascial remodeling at its finest. During some of my lectures I ask people to raise their hand if they have experienced or are experiencing just one of those issues. I usually get a 99 percent response in the affirmative. When I was younger, I used to get car sick, air sick, and sea sick really bad. It subsided as I got older, but then I started having problems with my muscles and joints by the age of 14 (My knees started hurting really bad). By the age of 22 I wrecked my back doing a deadlift, and by the time I was 32 I blew out my right knee. While I didn't understand what was going on with me, I accepted the consequences because I did lead an above average life of activity. I was destroying myself on a daily basis with running, weightlifting, and cycling! It wasn't until I fixed my atlas that the body aches and pain, as well as my motion sickness disappeared. Now that we have a grip on the situation, let's get to fixing yours!

The Muscles

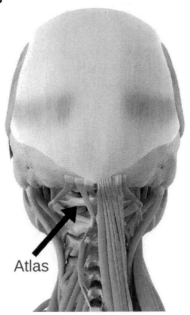
Atlas

      Most people will find out that their Atlas is offset primarily through visiting the chiropractor. The chiropractor will attempt to adjust it while very rarely achieving success. If the atlas does adjust, you can guarantee it will be maladjusted the very next day. This is because if you attempt to adjust the actual atlas vertebrae without relaxing the muscles surrounding it, the muscles will pull it back out of alignment through your normal function and body movements. When the atlas tilts, the small muscles surrounding it spasm and lock in order to stabilize the area. These are the muscles we are dealing with:

1. Obliquus Capitis Superior
2. Rectus Capitis Posterior Major
3. Obliquus Capitis Inferior
4. Intertransversarii Cervicis

Let's not forget that there are two sides to your neck, meaning eight very small, very strong muscles are spasming to lock down your skull, atlas, and axis. Having a chiropractor trying to adjust your atlas without first loosening up the surrounding tissue is like trying to open a door with a bazooka when it would be smarter to knock first. As you will see later, we actually get the muscles to straighten the atlas gently without the need for any popping and cracking.

So far we have three really serious problems. The first being our atlas is offset, compressing our brainstem. The second problem we have is that our very small, strong posterior neck muscles have gotten really tight, locking the area down. The third problem is the fact that all of this tightness compresses not only the brainstem, but nerves, and arteries that are surrounding and nourishing the area as well. When the atlas tilts and the head is crooked, the brain will make an autocorrection at the hips. This "shifting" of the hips will then make your head level at the cost of throwing your body into complete misalignment.

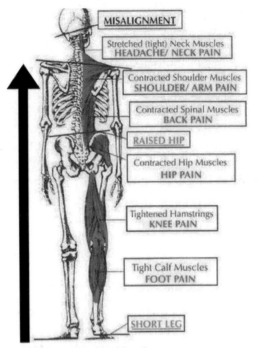

All of the muscles (Besides the neck) on this side of the body are stretched and get locked long in a state of anchored tension.

No one ever sees it coming – I sure didn't. This is a classic example of fascial remodeling, or the idea of the body being entirely connected. Rather than allow you to walk around with your head crooked, your brain contorts the rest of your body to make you feel balanced. You now function in dysfunction until your parts start wearing out – shoulder pain here, knee pain there, neck is stiff this day, then better the next. If you're an athlete you can run into some serious trouble, and it may even be a career ender. If you're a stay-at-home mom you'll just be wondering why you are feeling so old at such a young age.

If you look at the bottom of the previous picture, you will see that it states the end result of your atlas being off is a short leg. During my initial consultation the first thing I do is measure my clients feet, and nine out of 10 times I find a short leg, indicating a tilted/offset axis. When I show them how one foot is shorter than the other they always remark, "Yes I know, my chiropractor told me." I then ask if they tried to fix it and they always say, "Yes, they tried." This is proof once again that you cannot permanently fix a short leg through chiropractic. The short leg is a symptom. You don't cure a cold by treating a cough.

To fix the short leg, you must fix the atlas, but you must also relax the muscles on the tight side, and then relax the muscles on the stretched/anchored side. Because this is a book on upper body pain that is where we will concentrate.

Fixing The Problem

I realize that was a lot of information. You may be shaking your head like, "man, I bought the wrong book," but bear with me. I've been a coach for 20 years, and a great coach is a teacher first and an instructor second. I'm happy to let you know

I have ended my teaching portion for this book, and we are now getting into the instructing phase.

Fixing the atlas is simple – if I were to do it for you. I can typically align someones atlas in as little as five minutes. For you to do it manually, it is going to require a little more time and patience. You'll need to get a Back Buddy, which is a mobility tool for the head, neck, and upper back area. You can order one by going to my website www.chriskidawski.com

There is a reflexive point for the atlas right where your trapezius muscle meets your shoulder bone. By reflex I mean exactly what you are thinking. If I tap the front of your knee, your knee extends without you actively contracting your quadricep. By pressing into this reflex you will be releasing the small muscles surrounding your atlas.

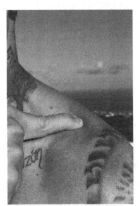

Using the correct knob on the Back Buddy and proper positioning is very important. You want to

use the pointy one on the side that has the larger loop.

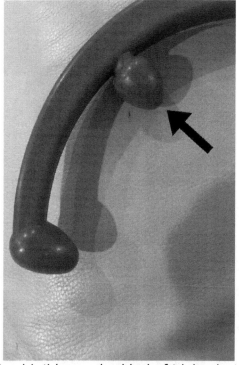

Like I said, this can be kind of tricky, but you will know when you hit the right spot because it will do three things:

1. Be very tender.
2. Open up pandora's box in your neck.
3. Send a tingling into the back of your head.

Please note some people do not experience any of those things, and some people experience more.

If I were to say the atlas were an enigma, that would be very kind of me!

To start the adjustment, you have to hook the Back Buddy behind your back, placing the knob in the area I showed you previously.

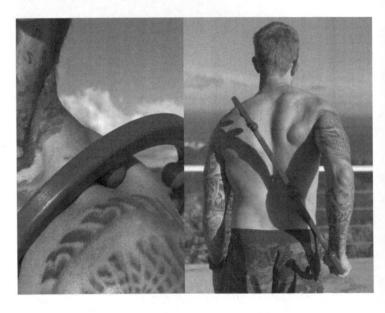

From that position you are going to pull down with the arm opposite the knob and lean forward, placing as much pressure on that reflex as you can.

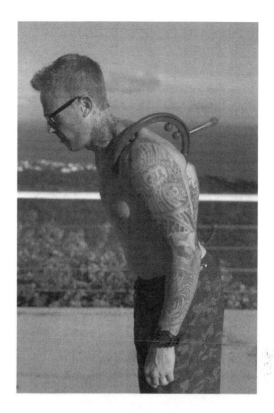

    Weird, I know. As far as I can find, there is no other documentation showing how to release the atlas reflex manually by yourself. In fact, I can't find anyone talking about the atlas reflex online except one other person right now, and the way he shows how to release it is very elementary, but at least he's on the right track.

    Typically you need to put pressure on the atlas reflex for around a minute per side. Doing each side four or five times per day should be enough to start. If you're not feeling what I'm describing, keep searching around in the area I reference, and I promise you'll find it. I have coached many people (through the computer even) to find their atlas reflex point – all it takes is a little determination and a lot of pressure. Don't give up!

The Mysteriously Elevated Shoulder

After applying pressure to your atlas reflex, I want you to look for a raised shoulder. If you look at yourself in the mirror this is what you should see.

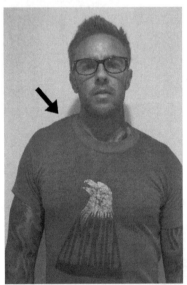

Whatever side is elevated is the short side of your neck, but the long side of the rest of your body needs to be released so your opposite side hip can drop down and relax. To do this you are going to sit down on the large loop of the Back Buddy on your opposite leg, and place the knob of the small loop on your trap muscle.

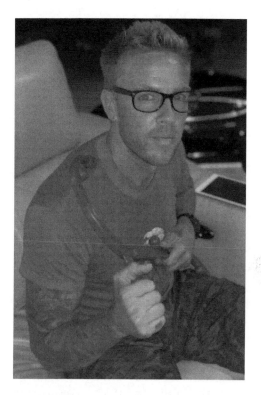

From there, rather than having to pull down quite hard and tire your arm out, you can just posture up to place sufficient pressure on your trap muscle. This muscle is tough, and you'll want to spend around 8-10 minutes penetrating the tissue to get it loose. Look for anything tender, tight, or sore. Please note that the shoulder will not drop overnight. You will probably need a month or two of working on it at least five times a week depending on how badly elevated your shoulder is till you start to see results. An extremely elevated shoulder like the one I show in the picture is one tough cookie. Be patient.

Last, But Not Least

Remember those small little muscles I was talking about earlier? Obliquus Capitis Superior and friends? Well these guys need some serious love now that we took the tourniquet off of your atlas with the last two mobilizations we did. There are two ways you can grind these guys out: the nice way or the easy way.

The Nice Way

To massage these guys the nice way, you'll want to use the two side by side knobs on the large loop of the Back Buddy. Put a little lotion on the back of your neck before you start, and then put both knobs on the back of your neck and slide them up and down applying as much pressure as you need to get a response.

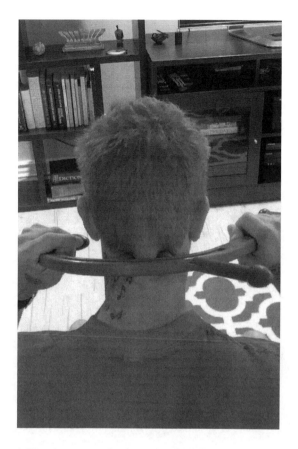

    I like to spend about 4-6 minutes gliding both of those knobs up and down my entire neck. In some instances, I will pin the tissue down in my neck and turn my head a couple of times to tear apart and unlock the small muscles that may be stuck.

The Easy Way

This way is a bit more intense because the circumference of the knob is a lot smaller, allowing for deeper penetration. To do this mobilization you are going to use the smallest knob on the shaft and grind into those small neck muscles right alongside your spine. Make sure to put lotion on your skin again.

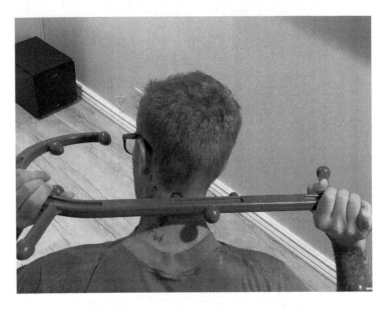

This technique is going to take a little longer, but not by much, because I am going to make you do each side for four minutes. Simply glide the little knob up and down, searching for tender or sore tissue. Please be careful – if your neck is really tight and you have never used anything to massage it before, this can be quite painful.

Surprisingly, that is it for the atlas. Now that you have started to get the atlas back in its home, the rest of the body will start shifting in your favor, moving back to true alignment. Working on the rest of your upper body will now be easier and more productive.

Opening up the atlas is a behemoth. I've had a lot of people experience a lot of interesting things with this mobilization. Numbness and tingling in the extremeties, fatigue, dizziness, nausea, on and off headaches, and difficulty sleeping. The benefits greatly outweigh all of the trouble, though, as your body starts to unwind itself, and the small aches and pains start to subside. The big aches and pains are going to require a little more attention, and that is where we are heading to next!

Ask The Coach: Are You a Chiro Hater, Or What?

I thought you would never ask, and the answer is no. My beef with their service is two-fold, though. First, they really do feel like they can fix all back problems, but as I have stated many times over in my Back Pain Bible book – back pain, a lot of times, is a symptom, not a problem. Second, people think that chiropractors can fix any and all back pain, and they get frustrated when they don't. There have been many times my clients have talked poorly about chiropractors and I stepped in to their defense, telling them the problem they have going on in their body can not be solved by chiropractic work, and reminding them that it's the medical system's fault for not being educated properly to help the people when they need it.

In fact, I just went to go see a chiropractor the other day to help me fix an issue I had going on that my methods were unable to correct. I didn't have any pain, but I could tell when I did some movements in the gym that my left arm was acting funny. When I pressed overhead, it felt like my left arm was crooked. I was also having difficulty taking a deep breath, and my diaphragm was getting locked up from time to time, even feeling bruised after doing endurance work. Rolling and stretching was not doing anything to alleviate the issues so I made an appointment with my chiropractor.

Within the first minute of being on the table my chiropractor found the problem. My first thoracic vertebrae was rotated. As he pressed on it a nervous shock was sent around both sides of my ribs ending in my diaphragm. If that wasn't weird enough, he found that my three cervical vertebrae (C3, C4, C5) were rotated as well, but in the opposite direction! This issue was distorting the signal my phrenic nerve was sending, which is responsible for you guessed it – the movement of my diaphragm. I have no idea how this happened, but this is a case where someone would be a candidate for spinal manipulation. My chiro adjusted me, and I went on my merry way.

The next day I went to the gym, and as soon as I put the bar over my head I felt 100 percent straight again – I knew the problem was fixed. One key aspect of going to see the chiropractor is to make sure you do soft tissue work before and after you see him or her. I did an hour of mobility before, and about 30 minutes after. Amazingly, minutes after being adjusted, my body told me where it went wrong. My left trapezius muscle instantly decided to lock up on me. When I got home I used the Back Buddy to loosen it up and boy did it ever feel amazing.

I realize you may be confused as to how I know all that, but you need to understand your body always wants to be in balance and will send you signals when things start to get out of whack. The problem is most people ignore those signals, pushing through whatever activity they are enjoying at the time. This is a recipe for disaster, and hopefully you will change your thinking after you read this book.

Chapter 2: Birds of a Feather Flock Together – Head & Neck Pain

Carlos was 27 years old and had been having debilitating migraines for the last 10 years of his life. The worst one he ever had put him out of commission in bed for nearly nine days. The problem was not the migraine, he said, it was the fact that he could literally "feel" it coming on, and the anxiety he would get was terrible.

During our first appointment, he commented that whenever he held something over his head his right shoulder would pinch really bad. Hearing this I went straight for his scalene muscles and as I palpated them, he nearly dropped to the floor. Carlos could not believe how sore those muscles were. I told him that I see this all the time in people that are in his profession – the IT business – because they are literally staring at the computer screen all day long with their shoulders raised, punching the keyboard.

I showed Carlos how to loosen them up with the Thera Cane. After five minutes of trying to do so, he was in an all out sweat. His eyes were blood shot, and he wanted to vomit from the pain. I asked him if those were the symptoms he would experience when getting a migraine, and he replied in the affirmative. After three days of doing the mobilization, Carlos said it felt like someone had taken a vice grip off of his head. It has been five years and what once was commonplace for Carlos is no longer even a concern. And if he ever does feel a little headache coming on he knows exactly what to do to stop it in its tracks!

Your Angry Muscle Tissue

I may have mentioned them once or twice already, and you may have even heard of them before, but to many people trigger points are still very much a mystery. To the medical field this is all hogwash as it is much easier (and more profitable) to prescribe you a pill, give you a shot, or cut you, then it is to teach you how to roll on a softball. Pills, shots, and surgery make great repeat customers as well.

Let me assure you trigger points are very real. I have felt my fair share in my body alone, let alone the bodies of all the clients I treat. In many ways, trigger points are the Bermuda Triangle of the pain world. You have primary trigger points, secondary trigger points, satellite trigger points, and latent trigger points. The network goes on and on. But by determining the causes of your trigger points, we can better map a path to treatment.

The primary causes for trigger points are:

- Psychological stress
- Mechanical stress

- Nutritional deficiencies
- Metabolic and endocrine inadequacies
- Visceral disease
- Infections and infestations

That's pretty broad, right? Sometimes it feels like just being alive can be a trigger point cause. A housewife who has never lifted weights could be in as much pain from a trigger point as an NFL lineman. These things are that vicious.

Trigger points can develop for a number of reasons, but for the purpose of this book we are going to focus more on the mechanical side. I'm willing to bet that if I assessed you, I would find that your pain is due to a movement/postural error.

As far as the different types of trigger points – this is where things can get a little like the tea cup ride at Disney World. But I should actually tell you what they are first.

Trigger points are little balls of ticked-off muscle tissue. When mechanical stress occurs on the same portion of tissue for too long, the muscle will actually spiral itself into a little ball. You can feel these suckers when you press into the tissue – they are like little pebbles. When the muscle spirals up it creates a compressive atmosphere that results in three things we don't want:

1. It chokes off its own blood supply, not letting any nutrients in.
2. It doesn't allow metabolic waste out from muscle energy production.
3. It changes the angle of pull of the muscle when it contracts, which will destabilize joints upstream and downstream from where it is located.

Inside this ball of tissue is a bunch of neurons that abide by one rule: "misery loves company." The tighter the ball gets, the more the neurons get compressed. And the more pissed off they become, they send pain to all areas of the body as an S.O.S. We, of course, politely ignore this most of the time.

Primary trigger points are the granddaddy problem makers. Finding and releasing them is tough, but when you do you can decrease your pain by 50 to 80 percent. I'm speaking from personal experience. Once I was unable to run for 10 days after releasing a trigger point in my groin muscle. My leg was incredibly sore the entire time, but my knee pain was drastically reduced. I had partially released a primary trigger point, but there was a secondary trigger point nagging my legs. Secondary trigger points will only be completely released if you release the primary trigger. I call these guys the cockroaches. You release it, and then four days later it pops back up again, and so the cycle begins.

Satellite trigger points develop as a result of the primary trigger, but are not directly connected. Because of this, I call these guys the "party crashers." Nobody invited them, but they'll be damned if some other trigger points are going to have fun without them. After releasing the primary trigger, you have to play seek and destroy with these guys to make sure the entire muscle (and fascia) is clear. Latent trigger points are a bit like a lone wolf combined with a sleepy dwarf. They have no reason to exist, and they do not refer pain, yet they are there. If you find one, you can easily get rid of it, which allows us to chalk up a big fat zero in the pain management game, but still can make us feel like we won.

Fibrosis, or fibrotic tissue, is defined by the overgrowth, hardening, and/or scarring of various tissues and is attributed to excess deposition of extracellular matrix components, including collagen. Fibrosis is the end result of chronic inflammatory reactions induced by a variety of stimuli, including persistent infections, autoimmune reactions, allergic responses, chemical insults, radiation, and tissue injury. When muscle tissue is fibrotic, it will feel like a long hard cable stuck in your body.

When I work with people, many ask how I always know exactly where the pain is. This is because muscles tell a story, and fibrosis is how it speaks. From a health perspective, muscle should be soft and supple, not hard and restricted. Fibrotic muscle tissue does not release – it breaks up very, very slowly, usually under the care of a very skilled body worker, as its sheaths become "unglued." I am working on developing a product that actually mimics a practitioner's forearm, allowing laypeople to once again become their own best therapists. Please sign up for my newsletter if you are interested in keeping abreast on this issue.

Rubbing EASE Magnesium spray into fibrotic muscle tissue will help erode any calcium deposits that have formed on or around the muscle tissue. We have four neurotransmitters in the body. They are potassium (excitable), sodium (excitable), calcium (excitable), and magnesium (calming). Did you get that? You have three neurotransmitters responsible for exciting your nervous system, and one that is responsible for calming it down. Over 75 percent of the U.S. population is deficient in magnesium because it is no longer present in sufficient amounts in our soil. We've known this since 1923. Yep.

Before a muscle becomes fibrotic, it gets stuck in a tonic state, producing a continuous contraction that calls upon copious amounts of calcium to sustain it. Because the muscle is so tense, it operates on the same principles as trigger points trapping the metabolic waste in the muscle tissue. When enough waste builds up, you get a calcium crust that forms around it, making it harder and harder. If you have a poor diet this can happen even quicker. When treating fibrotic tissue, you must be the stoic one. I have worked on fibrotic tissue of my own for over a year before it finally broke up. I was not sad to see it go.

Adhesions are primarily made from myofibroblasts and are a whole different beast. Myofibroblasts are large cells with ruffled membranes and highly active endoplasmic reticulum (the outside of their cells do stuff). They possess bundles of microfilaments, which terminate at the cell surface in a specialized adhesion complex, termed the fibronexus or mature local adhesion. Myofibroblasts migrate to and are highly responsive to chemokines released at the site of injury. In short, these guys attract white blood cells, telling your body you are hurt. Interestingly, these guys add a rogue contraction property to the fascial net I keep talking about. Under certain conditions (say trauma, like a Charlie horse or pulled hamstring) these fibroblasts hook their cellular structure into the connective tissue matrix and then exert a slow smooth muscle-like contraction into the fibrous webbing. Think of it as Velcro with a mind of its own, reaching out and playing with your fascia at will.

Adhesions need cross-friction, vibration, and in some cases just good old smashing to break them up. They are especially prevalent around injury sites such as pulls, strains, and sprains, as well as surgical incisions.

Why cover all of this stuff? Because I have seen that a majority of pain in the upper body is referred by trigger points or adhesions that are not allowing your muscles to work correctly. For instance, I have people coming to me for shoulder pain every single week, yet I have them working in many other areas, never once touching their actual shoulder. This is because we have 15 muscles that surround the shoulder to help it function the way it is supposed to. For pain to develop in the shoulder, I find typically between three and five of those muscles have developed trigger points or adhesions. You feel the pain in your shoulder, but your brain feels the pain in the muscles that *support* the shoulder. As I said in the introduction, this is what makes pain in the upper body so dang difficult to solve – it hides very well, and is very deceptive.

Let's throw a monkey wrench into their tomfoolery.

Masters of Chaos – The Scalenes

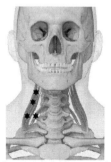

The black stars are trigger point locations

The scalenes make me mad. How mad you ask? I have to put these muscles in the neck pain section even though they don't refer pain into the neck! The scalenes are like the Mariana Trench in the pacific ocean. The Mariana Trench is more than 36,000 feet deep and god knows what lives down there. I say this because when you start poking around the scalenes you have no idea what you are going to find.

The scalenes have a very important job, though, and that is why I am going over them first here. If you look at where they originate, and where they insert, you'll notice that these muscles are the prime movers of the head and actually relate the position of your head back to the brain. The dizziness you feel on a boat or a rollercoaster – that's your scalenes not being able to keep up with the change of direction they are experiencing. Besides motion sickness, the scalenes (in conjunction with an offset atlas) are responsible for the feeling of vertigo, as well as sending a tremendous amount of pain down the arm, into the chest, and into the upper portion of your back between your shoulder blades. This all happens from the development of trigger points in them.

When scalenes get tight they pull the first rib up, pinching your median nerve that runs down the arm all the way to the fingers. This will result in not only pain, but weakness in that arm as well. When we go to the doctor describing pain in the shoulder or arm, they try to treat the arm with minimal results. When we go to physical therapy with pain in our shoulder or arm, they give you shoulder and arm exercises. Here's a muscle geek tip for you, when a muscle is short and tight, it is chronically contracted. When you have a chronically contracted muscle, the last thing you want to do is contract it some more!

Below is a graphic of the areas scalene trigger points can send pain to in your body:

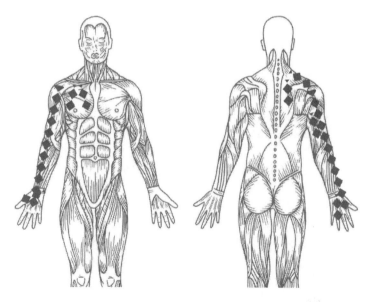

The red shaded areas indicate pain.

Like I said, these guys really are that bad. Anterior (front) shoulder pain is the worst pain I find the trigger points in the scalenes will create. We will revisit this in the anterior shoulder pain section, but for now just keep a mental note of it.

As you can tell by the client story at the beginning of this chapter releasing the scalenes is not the most fun thing to do with your time. If you are experiencing any of the symptoms I spoke of, then it becomes an essential thing to do with your time, though. Before we get down to the nitty gritty I would like to extend a word of caution. There is a massive network of nerves, lymph nodes, and blood vessels that span the entire portion of your neck that we will be digging in when trying to release the scalenes. I was taught in school, and in my specialized certifications that going into the scalenes is a no-no. I was told it's dangerous and as a therapist you do so at your own peril because if you hit one of these nerves/blood vessels/lymph nodes you could seriously harm your client.

Having said that, I have been digging in peoples scalenes, and having them dig in their own for the last 12 years, and I have never once injured someone, nor have I had someone injure themselves. In fact, people only get better. The old saying goes, "To get somewhere you have never gotten before, you have to do something you've never done before." In other words, you must be a pioneer with your pain. The trick (read obvious thing to do) with this mobilization is to start off light; very light even. The trigger points will feel like little bumps in your neck, and if the pain starts travelling down your arm, or into the area that feels painful, then you've found one. You're in the right area.

To start, rub a little lotion on the side of the neck you are going to work on. Then, place the large loop of the Back Buddy under your leg to keep it upright and stable. Use the round knob extending from the back buddy to put pressure on your scalenes, then glide on the muscle from your collar bone to the base of your skull.

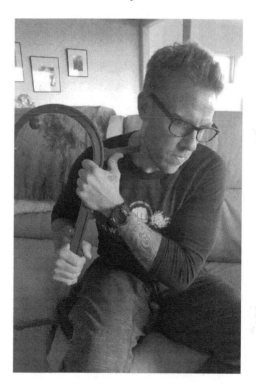

Glide on the tissue for 4-6 minutes at a time. When you finish, it's time to stretch the tight side to open it up further. To do this you are going to sit down in something like a dinner table chair. Grab underneath the chair with the hand of the tight side we are going to stretch. Next grab your head with the opposite hand and pull your head away from your hand until you feel a pretty good stretch. Hold the stretch for 20-30 seconds and then rest. Repeat that stretch 4-5 times, or until you feel like you made a decent change to the tissue.

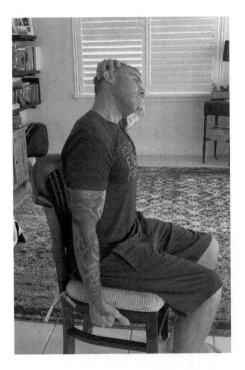

The Sternocleidomastoid (SCM)

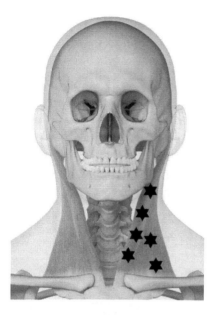

Though it looks big and bad, the SCM is honestly a gentle giant. The most identifiable muscle in the neck, all you have to do is turn your head to see it sticking out. I'm grouping this muscle in with the scalenes because you are going to mobilize it the same way. In fact – you already have. As you can see by the illustration, there are plenty of trigger points sitting in this muscle, most of which refer pain into the back of the head and around the eyes.

The trigger points will present themselves as little bumps, or hard pieces of tissue. Pressing on them with the Thera Cane, or Back Buddy should reproduce the same pain you have when you get a headache. Be gentle with them – if they are bad enough, they will leave you a little disoriented after you get done playing with them. These muscles also tell the brain where the head is located. Any dizziness that occurs as a result of applying pressure into the muscles to release the tissue should be expected and can last for up to 45 minutes. I find that resting on the couch or bed with your head in a stable, comfortable position helps while everything gets calibrated again. Avoid having your head tilted to one side.

The Trapezius

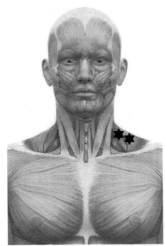

Affectionately called the "traps" by all the bros in every gym in America, these guys are not comprised of the cute little muscles you see in the diagram above. Rather, they are actually a very large sheet of muscle tissue that makes up a huge piece of your back tissue. Starting in your lower thoracic spine region, this muscle connects to the back of your head. The reason why I only show you the cute little part is because that is where some of your monstrous head and neck pain can be residing. When the traps get tight they will pull down on the back of the neck causing your scalenes and SCM to work harder to keep the head level. If the traps get really bad, they can even contribute to back pain.

Your traps are your workhorse. Anytime you get stressed whether in the office, in traffic, or at home, these guys suffer. If you've ever been in a car accident, I can guarantee your traps are damaged heavily, and have developed trigger points as a result. With the amount of time spent at computers these days people's posture will suffer. Typing, or simply sitting with your arms outstretched, can call on the trapezius muscle to stay elevated for hours at a time. After years of this abuse we wonder then, why we get headaches, or why our traps are so tight.

You can walk around the mall, go to the beach, or walk around the park and I guarantee you will see someone touching, rubbing, or sometimes downright yanking on this area of their body. Others will resort to Advil, or other over-the-counter medication to alleviate the stress. Rather than resort to half measures, I'm going to show you how to release them correctly – for good.

Starting off, you are going to once again put the larger of the two openings under the opposite leg of the trap you are working on so the Back Buddy crosses your body. You can place the knob directly on the trap and pull down, but I find that wastes a lot of energy. As you place the knob of the small opening into the area of your trap that is shown to have the trigger point in it, all you have to do is posture up from there and let gravity do the work.

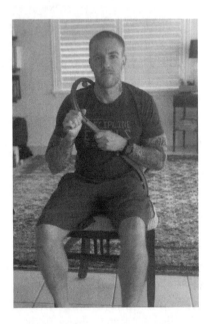

Do not underestimate the tenderness of these muscles. I have had people forget their own name when mobilizing this trigger point – they can be that nasty. I also like to search around a bit, and I have often found some strings, or other little bumps, hiding in there that were referring pain into my head. The traps can be very tough to break up so be consistent in showing them some love, especially if you have a desk job or are stressed out on the regular.

The Levator Scapulae

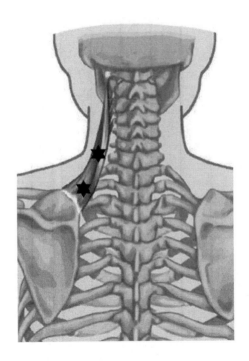

If the traps are the workhorses, then the levator scapulae is the workhorse behind the workhorse. The reason why: levator scapulae do just as much work as the traps do with 1/10th as much muscle. Once again, and at the cost of sounding like a broken record, this muscle is heavily abused if you sit and work at a computer all day. Levator scapulae does exactly what it sounds like it does – it pulls your shoulders up to your ears. If we lead a very stressed out life at work, in traffic, at home, heck if we even carry our purse on the same shoulder or pin the phone between our ear and shoulder for too long, this little guy will suffer big time.

There are two trigger points in this muscle that cause it to get short and tight, which then refers a lot of pain up into the head. When this happens, we unknowingly reach for the pain medication, masking the real issue at hand. This guy is not going to be the walk in the park it looks like. I had to release mine on my right shoulder one time, and it was so tender it nearly made me black out.

The pain these trigger point can cause will be debilitating at times, travelling up the back of the neck, going behind the ear, pushing through the temple before it stops right behind the eye. Mobilizing this little beast can cause you to literally feel like your eye is going to pop out of its socket. Rest assured it will not.

To start, place the large opening over your shoulder and utilize the pointy knob that is at the end. Place the tip of the knob on the top of your scapula and pull your arms down to apply pressure. If the tissue is tender, sore, or referring pain you hit the jackpot. If you are not feeling anything, search around to make sure the area is clear before giving up too fast.

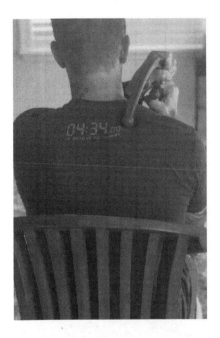

Pain from the levator scapula can also be referred into the shoulder as well as between your shoulder blades. If you are experiencing pain in these areas there is no harm in applying some pressure on those muscles with the same knob while you are back there.

The second trigger point is going to be a little bit more challenging to release, but is a must if your neck has been stiff or you are getting headaches in your temples or behind your eyes. You're looking for the area where your trap and your neck connect (please refer to the previous picture). Place the knob at the end of the smaller opening of the Back Buddy right where your trap connects with your neck and see if there is anything sketchy in the area. When you find a little bump, or some patchy tissue, pull your arms down to apply pressure. From there you can tilt your head away from the Back Buddy to the opposite shoulder. This will stretch the area and with luck break apart the trigger point in the process.

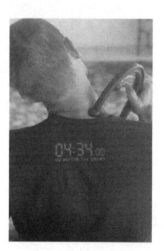

You may have to repeat the tilting of the head several times before the trigger lets go. To picture this think of breaking a paper clip. You'll never break a paper clip by bending it one time; you have to bend it several times before the metal breaks. Focus on tilting your head away, then bringing it back several times while pinning the tissue down. Lift the knob up off of your skin and place it in a different area from time to time to make sure you are releasing all of the fibrotic tissue.

The Rhomboids

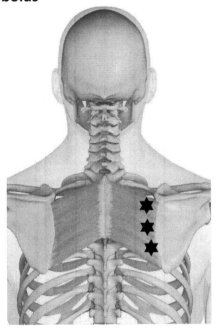

Loosening up the rhomboids can make it feel like an elephant just jumped off of your shoulders. This muscle is responsible for pinching your shoulder blades together as if you were trying to puff out your chest. They also help rotate your shoulder and elevate it as well. Poor posture, not overwork, often leads to pain in this area. When we sit with our shoulders rounded forward and our back hunched, our rhomboids get locked in a stretched position, which puts a lot of stress on them at their shoulder blade attachment sites. Trigger points develop and refer pain into the area, which people will complain about then largely ignore. The pain is there to do two things: to tell you to stop hunching and to call you to put pressure in the area to maintain the health of the tissue.

To open the rhomboids up you are going to have to tape two lacrosse balls together or purchase a specially made ball for this exercise from my website www.chriskidawski.com If the lacrosse balls are too painful for you, then start the exercise off with two tennis balls taped together. Rather than teach through pictures for this mobilization, I recorded a YouTube video. Go to https://youtu.be/USA_m1qZhPI to check it out. If it works for you, please give me a thumbs up. Also, if you have any comments, post them below the video, and I'll get back to you pronto!

The Splenius Muscles

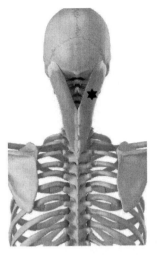 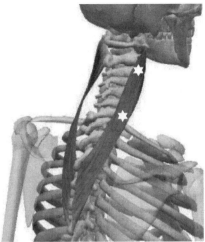

Splenius Capitis   Splenius Cervicis

The splenius muscles extend the cervical portion of your spine and flex and rotate your head to the same side. Think for a second about how often you rotate your head every day. What about if you sleep wrong? Everyone in the world has woken up at least once with a kink in his or her neck. Most of us just deal with that pesky kink until it goes away, very rarely seeking out treatment.

Because these muscles are connected from your spine to your skull (capitis), and your spine to your atlas and axis (cervicis), when trigger points develop the muscle will get short and tight, pulling down and back on the skull and tugging on that atlas/axis connection. With those connection points being stressed it's no surprise that these two muscles will serve up a generous portion of neck and head pain.

Thankfully the trigger points for these muscles are in an easy enough spot to work out. To do this mobilization, you are going to once again use the two knobs that are side by side on the large opening of the Back Buddy. Put a little lotion on the back of your neck and then place one knob on each side, gliding up and down as you search for any bumps or tender tissue.

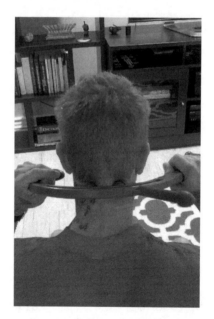

Work the tissue for between four and six minutes, pressing a little deeper as the time progresses. Please note that your spine is right in between both of those knobs. I like to turn and twist the Back Buddy in order to get to some tender tissue if I have to, but you do not want to grind on your spine!

That concludes the portion of this book on head and neck pain. I'm going to say it again – your biggest challenge/goal is to get that atlas/axis relationship corrected. If you're not making any headway with the mobility exercises, it may be a good idea for you to go see a chiropractor who specializes in atlas correction. Call around and see what you find. If you do not correct your atlas first, then you need to get into the flow of maintaining a head/neck pain-treatment regimen because I have found every single pain in the upper body starts with that vertebrae being out of place. Now, on to the shoulders!

Ask the Coach: Do You Recommend a Specific Pillow?

While there is special consideration for people who have neck pain upon rising from their slumber, I do not recommend and specific type of pillow. While getting a pillow specific to your style of sleeping (Side, back, stomach) is better than just any old pillow, I tell people that you should train yourself to sleep on your back, especially if you are an athlete. The reason why most people can't fall asleep and stay asleep is two-fold. First approximately 90 percent of people in the world lack sufficient amounts of magnesium to help relax us when the time comes. The second thing is that people do not put themselves in a restful position to sleep when they lay down.

In Esther Gokhale's book *8 Steps To A Pain Free Back,* she discusses how she studied an African tribe that had no incidences of back pain at all. Her finding showed that they slept on their backs on the ground and their spine actually developed a J curve instead of the traditional S curve anatomy books show. Her recommendations are to sleep on your back with a pillow under your lower leg, and your shoulders and head on your pillow.

I was the world's greatest side sleeper, and surprise, surprise, I always had disrupted sleep accompanied by minor neck issues. When I became strict with her recommendations, my neck issues slowly started to disappear and my sleep dramatically improved. Sleeping on my back is the primary way I sleep now, with only occasional side sleeping. This is another win in the posture category and goes to show you can't just buy some new gadget, the latest pillow, or take copious amounts of melatonin in order to sleep. You need to orient your body correctly and let gravity do the rest. If you would like help achieving optimal rest, please go to my website and click on "Chris Approved Supplements" and navigate to the sleep section where you will find all of my little secrets to sleep and recover better.

Chapter 3: Where Your Shoulder Pain Is Really Coming From

Julie was a competetive CrossFitter with a propensity for pushing through the pain. Everyone marvelled at her work ethic and strength – a perfect combination for her sport. What everyone didn't know was that her left shoulder was killing her. Rather than skip upper body exercises or scale to a lighter weight, she kept her foot on the gas, giving every workout her all.

One day during a competition Julie was performing muscle-ups on the rings when her worst nightmare came true. She heard a crunch in her shoulder, and as she came down from the rings a nice loud pop occurred. She was in incredible pain, unable to even lift up her arm. A trip to the doctor the next day confirmed a torn rotator cuff muscle in her left shoulder, but all Julie heard was that the doctor thought she will most likely never CrossFit again in her life. Julie broke down crying like a baby and seriously felt like her life was over.

Julie heard of me from a friend of a friend. Figuring anything was better than surgery and never CrossFitting again, she set up an appointment and gave me a try. During the assessment, her shoulder sounded like it was a non-stop popcorn-popping machine. Any time she moved it there were pops, cracks, and snaps. When I asked her how long her shoulder had been bothering her before it exploded, she told me about two years. Two years is an eternity when it comes to the shoulder.

Clearly seeing that her range of motion in that shoulder was suffering, I immediately had her roll out her subscapularis muscle. As soon as she got into it she forgot all about her shoulder pain and became consumed with how tender that muscle was. Other areas we needed to correct were the rotator cuff and lat. It took three months, but Julie finished the program and now had zero pain in her shoulder – all without going under the knife. She was very thankful for the help, and still does CrossFit to this day. My one demand before she left was that she speak up a lot sooner if anything started to hurt again!

It's Not Me, It's You

My friend who is a physical therapist was talking to me about the shoulder and described it in such a beautiful way that I teach it to every single one of my shoulder pain clients still to this day. He said, "Everyone thinks the shoulder is a ball and socket joint, but the fact that it can be repeatedly dislocated and reset shows that it is not a true ball and socket. The shoulder is actially more like a softball sitting on a golf tee."

That statement about a softball sitting on a golf tee is what I see when I get shoulder pain clients. The fact of the matter is (and I hate speaking in absolutes) in 12 years I have never treated a persons shoulder for shoulder pain. Shoulder pain once again is a symptom not a problem. If you treat the shoulder you will keep treating it until you are blue in the face.

There are 15 (yes 15) muscles that surround the shoulder helping it function and stay in place. The trapezius, levator scapulae, and rhomboids originate from the base of the skull and/or spine and connect the scapula (your shoulder wing) and clavicle to the trunk of your body. The pectoralis major, pectoralis minor, latissimus dorsi, teres major and deltoid connect to the top end of the humerus (upper arm bone) and anchor it to the body. There are four rotator cuff muscles - the subscapularis, supraspinatus, infraspinatus and teres minor, which connect the scapula to the humerus and provide support for the glenohumeral joint, (where the softball sits on the golf tee). The last three muscles are flexors and extensors of the arm and include the biceps, triceps, and a funny-looking (and sounding) muscle called the coracobrachialis.

When someone has shoulder pain, I typically find they have a problem with at least 3-5 of the 15 muscles, sometimes more. Clearing up the shoulder pain is as easy as finding out which muscles are tight, or laden with trigger points, and then releasing them. To do this we have to do a little bit of seeking and destroying, but it can be done and done quite easily for that matter.

Front of the Shoulder Pain

Rotator Cuff Muscles

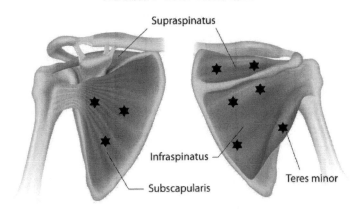

Anterior view   Posterior view

Anterior means front, posterior means back.

Pictured above are your rotator cuff muscles. These guys get used and abused to the max, especially if your are in a throwing sport. Bad falls can extensively damage the rotator cuff muscles as well. If you're involved in any type of weightlifting, especially powerlifting, I can almost guarantee the pain in the front of your shoulder that you continuously ignore is coming from one of these four muscles. The reason these muscles get so abused is because they are responsible for slowing your arm down after that 98 mile an hour pitch, literally brace all of your bodyweight when you plant your hand as you are falling, and are responsible for stabilizing that 400 some odd pounds you try to bench press every Monday. Simply put, they are very small, but have very big, heavy jobs to do.

When people are told they have a rotator cuff issue, I usually see them break out some bands or do rotator cuff exercises with dumbbells. While this may work okay for some people, it gets most of us in even more trouble. Did you see all of the trigger points that can develop in these four muscles? All of that pain goes to one area – the front part of your shoulder. Luckily, relief is not too far off if you know where to look, which is exactly what I'm going to teach you.

The Infraspinatus

Located smack dab on your shoulder blade, loosening up this part of your rotator cuff is like sticking bamboo shoots under your fingernails. The pain can be sharp and surprising when you apply pressure. Think of it this way: it's communicating how angry it is with you for not taking care of it for so long. To relax the tissue in this muscle apply pressure in the areas where the trigger points reside with the pointy knob located on the end of the large opening on the Back Buddy. You'll know when you find a spot -- it will be sharp and alarming.

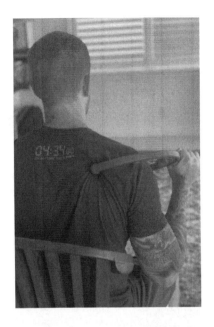

Go slow and be curious. Search the entire shoulder blade applying pressure to anything you feel is sore, especially if it is referring pain into the front part of the shoulder. I like to work this area for between 4 and 6 minutes or until it is so tender I am forced to stop. Because of how tight this muscle gets and how musch tension it can hold, do not be surprised if the muscle feels bruised the next day. If it is pat yourself on the back (avoiding your shoulder blade of course) because that means you relieved some tension or broke up a trigger point.

The Supraspinatus

A much smaller muscle than the infraspinatus, this guy can still pack quite a wallop in the pain department. This muscle is located right on top of your shoulder blade and will be released much in the same way as you released your trap muscle. Grab your Back Buddy. Using the knob at the end of the smaller opening, apply downward pressure into the top of your shoulder blade.

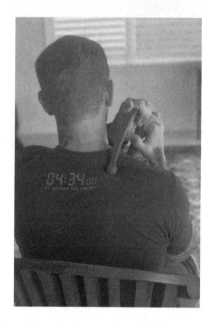

Search from the end closest to your spine, moving out to the edge of your shoulder in a slow patient manner for 4-6 minutes, digging into any areas that are sore, tender, tight, or referring pain into the front part of the shoulder. This muscle breaks up rather quickly, and I really haven't had too many cases of it being sore after. Be consistent with your approach to helping it get better.

The Teres Minor

If the infraspinatus feels like bamboo shoots, this guy is reminiscent of driving an ice pick into your back. When this muscle gets tight it refers pain into the front part of your shoulder, and it will also pinch down on your tricep tendon, shortening it and creating pain all the way down the back of your arm. There was a chiropractor in Hawaii I would go to when I was younger that always worked on this muscle for me because he knew I used to be a pitcher in high school. The pain was both alarming and euphoric, and I quickly developed a love/hate relationship with releasing it.

To get at this muscle we are going to use a lacrosse ball. Once again, I shot a video for you so you can better understand how to open this muscle up. If this is an e-book, just click on the link, if you are reading a paperback please type the following URL into your browser:

https://youtu.be/ORRjaW3NqjU

The Subscapularis

The transmittal of pain from this muscle eluded me for years, until I had to release it on myself. Your subscapularis muscle is a thick piece of muscle tissue that sits on the inside of your shoulder blade. If you were to look into a mirror and raise your arm up, it would be staring right at you from your arm pit. If you bench press heavy, this muscle is helping to lower and stabilize the weight, as well as press it back up. If you do CrossFit or Gymnastics and have pain when you are training on the rings, but not when you are training on anything else, then your subscap is tight and does not have the ability to expand. The pain you feel is your brain letting you know that muscle is in trouble and the movement you are doing is not safe.

The pain pattern this muscle produces is odd, and I liken it to a candy cane hanging on your arm with the stem going down into your bicep. When I palpate the front of the shoulder and the bicep of someone who has a tight subscap the tissue is thick and tight and quite painful. Because this is such a sensitive area of your body, I urge you to start off slow with the mobilization. Use a softball at first, then graduate to a baseball. If the softball is too harsh for you at the beginning, then lay on a foam roller. Because of the complexity of this exercise, I shot another video for you and posted it to youtube. To view it go to https://youtu.be/PLkXp4GJCt4.

The remaining portion of this section is devoted to muscles that cut off or restrict the brachial plexus and send pain into the front part of your shoulder or down your arm. The brachial plexus is a network of nerves the supply sensation to the skin and muscles going down your arm.

The Brachial Plexus

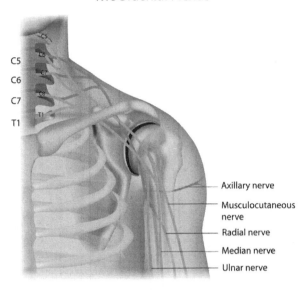

The reason why these muscles disrupt the nerves is because their attachments pass right on top of them. When they get tight, they will compress the nerve, causing pain.

The Scalenes

As I mentioned before, the scalenes will send a generous portion of pain down into the front part of the shoulder, and if they get tight enough – all the way down to the hand. Please refer back to the section on the scalenes to revisit how to loosen them up.

The Subclavius

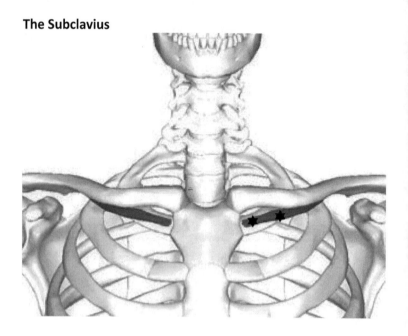

Moving from the sternum to the clavicle, this little muscle can cause big pain when it gets tight or develops trigger points. To compound that effect, the subclavian vein and subclavian artery run right underneath it as well.

The mobility exercise to release this muscle is actually quite easy. Starting off in a seated position you are going to hook the small opening of the Back Buddy under your leg. From there, angle the pointed knob directly under your clavicle and with a little bit of lotion applied grind back and forth from your sternum to your shoulder.

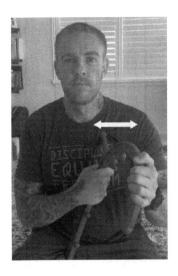

Do this for 1-2 minutes and look for hard tissue or any pain going down your arm.

Pec Major & Minor

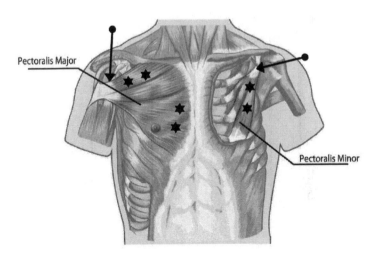

The stars represent trigger points, and the arrows represent where the brachial plexus gets pinched.

The pectoralis muscles (Pecs as the Bro's call them) are much more worrisome for the men than the women. There is one caveat for the women though – if you decide to get breast implants, you will want to mobilize your high pec quite a bit because I have seen the pec minor and major freeze on some women who have implants, creating an alarming amount of pain in the shoulder in the process. Guys will have trigger points develop in the pectoral muscles due to heavy and frequent bench pressing.

Mobilizing these muscles is easy. Grab a softball and find the corner of a wall in your home where you can apply pressure to your chest with the ball and stick your head through a little. With the ball pinned between the wall, and your chest, start rolling around the chest moving your arm out to the side.

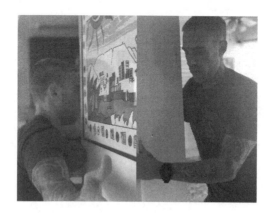

Do this mobilization for 4-6 minutes applying as much pressure as you feel is necessary to get the desired result. If you run into any knots feel free to pin them down and see if they refer pain into your shoulder - most likely they will. When the softball no longer refers any pain, use a baseball, or a baseball sized mobility ball I approve of from my website. The last step would be to use a lacrosse ball to really get into some tight corners and clear everything out.

The Biceps

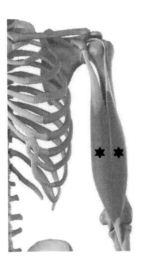

The biceps are pretty much everyone's favorite muscle. Look at any fitness magazine in the checkout aisle at your local supermarket and you'll see another shredded guy or girl flexing his or her bicep at you. In the bodybuilding world, the bicep is a popular elbow flexor (it bends your arm), but in my world the bicep is a misused and underappreciated shoulder extensor (It raises your arm) and stabilizer. This is what we are going to focus on here.

Think about how many times you bend your arm every day, and think about how many times you raise it. If you're a woman, think about how much you carry a purse with you arm locked out at 90 degrees stressing the bicep in an isometric fashion. Even though I'm putting this muscle at the last part of this section, do not underestimate the problems trigger points here can produce for the shoulder.

In order to open this muscle up, you'll want to use a lacrosse ball up against the wall at the edge of a corner again. Roll the ball from the elbow, to the shoulder and look for those two trigger points right in the belly of the muscle.

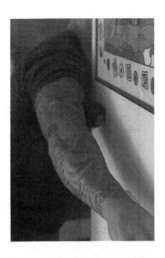

    I recommend rolling the bicep for 2-3 minutes in this fashion. If the lacrosse ball is too targeted, you can start off with a baseball or softball – both of which have a larger circumference and will cover more area.

    As a finisher, I highly recommend rolling the front part of the shoulder with a lacrosse ball up against the wall. Even though pain does not originate in that area, the pain trigger points refer into that area can stir things up a bit and cause a traffic jam in the fascia. I typically spend about 3 or 4 minutes in the area placing direct pressure, as well as rolling the ball up and down on the front delt to alleviate some of the stress that was caused.

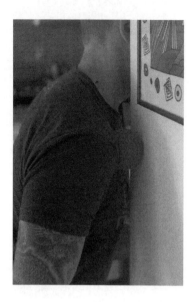

    I hope you enjoyed this portion of the book and discovered some pain points you never knew you had. Let's move on to the last portion now, where we traverse the world of rear delt pain!

Back of the Shoulder Pain

While much rarer in my opinion, pain at the back of the shoulder can still be pretty irritating, especially if you are a weightlifter or an athlete. The good news is that in my experience pain in the back of the shoulder is much easier to get rid of than pain in the front of the shoulder.

Several of the muscles we already worked on not only refer pain into the front of the shoulder, but into the back of the shoulder as well. These muscles are:

1. The Levator Scapulae (head & neck pain section).
2. The Supraspinatus (front of the shoulder pain section).
3. The Teres Minor (front of the shoulder pain section).
4. The Subscapularis (front of the shoulder pain section).
5. The Tapezius (head & neck pain section).

Please realize that it may not be just one of those muscles that is causing your pain but several. If you are unlucky enough to have a frozen shoulder, all five of those muscles may be on the fritz and causing your shoulder pain. Please reference back to those sections if the mobilizations that follow do not adequately target your back of the shoulder pain.

The Teres Major

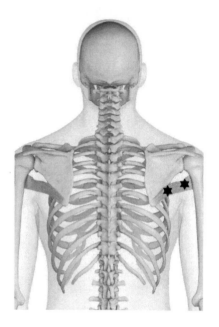

    The teres major muscle originates on your shoulder blade and attaches to your upper arm. The reason this guy will cause pain in the back of your shoulder is because your radial nerve, which exits your spine and travels down your arm, runs right under the teres minor. When the teres minor gets tight, it compresses that nerve and creates a world of hurt for you.

    Because this muscle can get super duper tender when it develops trigger points or gets tight, you'll want to start off the mobilization with something that has a larger circumference like a softball. Begin by laying on your side and placing the softball where your armpit meets your shoulder. If you have a problem there, you will already start to feel some pain. Then roll onto your back just a little bit to put more direct pressure onto the teres major. If the pain level is high congratulations – you have trigger points in there and that is where your pain is coming from.

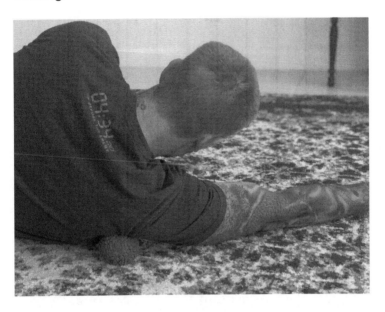

    The teres major tends to loosen up and get sore pretty quickly so I recommend only spending about 2-3 minutes rolling the ball around in there. If it's sore the next day or two leave it alone and then go back to it when you can comfortably apply pressure. As the muscle loosens up, the softball will no longer do the job. I recommend graduating to the baseball. The brave of heart can then tackle the lacrosse ball. If you can roll around on your teres major with a lacrosse ball without any pain, than she is free and clear, and you can move on to the next mobilization.

The Serratus Posterior Superior

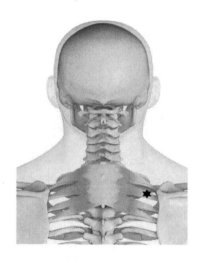

Looks pretty harmless, right? Guess again. If active, that little trigger point can destroy the function of your entire arm. This is one of those trigger points – like the ones in the scalenes – I just had to develop a pain pattern for in the body. Here it is:

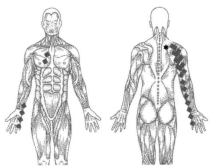

The black star is the trigger, shaded area is the pain pattern.

Okay, so you can see the damage it does to the back of the shoulder, all the way down the arm. It even gets the wrist and your poor little pinky. Did you notice the shaded area on the chest, though? That guy is the biggie.

Most people think we breathe with our lungs. However, our lungs are only the vessels by which breath takes place. I know what you are going to say next, "We actually breathe with our diaphragm" – and you'd be partly right. We do breathe with our diaphragm, but respiration would not occur if it were not for the pull of the following muscles:
1. The external intercostals
2. Intercostalis intimi
3. Subcostals
4. Sternocleidomastoid
5. Scalene muscles
6. Pec major and minor
7. Serratus anterior
8. Latissimus dorsi

9. Serratus posterior anterior
10. Serratus posterior superior
11. Iliocostalis cervicis
12. Rectus abdominis
13. External obliques
14. Internal obliques
15. Transverse abdominis
16. Serratus posterior inferior
17. Quadratus lumborum

If that list didn't shock you, here is an amazing diagram I found depicting the respiratory process from a muscle standpoint:

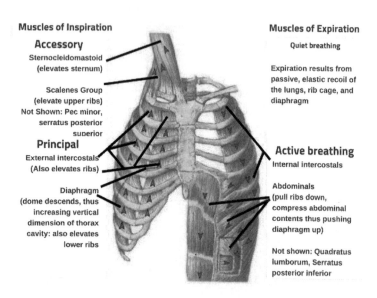

Respiration is initiated by the muscles, reinforced by the diapragm, and carried out by the lungs. Like I said earlier, the lungs are merely a vessel for the exchange of gases which keep us alive.

Somewhere in there you saw the serratus posterior superior muscle mentioned. This muscle expands the rib cage upon inhalation, and because about .01 percent of us breathe correctly, this muscle will develop a trigger point referring pain right into the lung area. This will automatically slow your breathing down and make you take it easier so you do not tax the muscle as much. Loosening it up is not that much of a chore. I shot a video a long time ago showing people how to mobilize it and in less than a year it has over 3,000 views! Please check it out on YouTube again here: https://youtu.be/jVGHIC0bYqo.

The Latissimus Dorsi

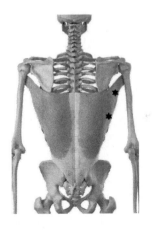

Your latissimus dorsi (or "lats" as the bros call them) are a massive slab of upper body muscle that play a huge part in how your shoulder and arm function during a myriad of activities. In the last section on the serratus posterior superior, we even noted that it is a contributor to respiration. What is even more shocking about this muscle is that it connects to such a low point on the spine that some coaches and physical therapists actually consider it to be a core muscle. They would be correct.

What fascinates me about the lats is that they are the only muscle in the human body that connect the shoulder to the hips. This makes them integral in how the legs and arms function in exercises like sprinting, rowing, and jumping – and you thought it was just used for pullups!

This mobilization is very intense, so I highly suggest starting off with a softer foam roller, then progressing to a firmer one. To start, lay down on your side with the roller tucked in where your shoulder and lat meet. From there you are going to grab your arm and pull it back behind you slightly. If that pressure is challenging for you then stay there. If not, you may raise your hip up off the ground and use your legs to pull yourself as you roll up and down the top half of your lats.

Again, this is a tough mobilization to depict in a picture, so I shot another video for you. Please check it out here: https://youtu.be/LHTv7ruO6-A.

Because the lats are so massive and so strong, I want you to camp out on this muscle for between 8 and 10 minutes. Doing this correctly will be gruelling but effective. I say 2-4 minutes in the video to start off with, but the best course of action would be to do 2-4 minutes for two sets, taking a 10 minute break in between. If you find any hot spots, don't hesitate to pin them down on the roller till they give up and relax. Try to pinpoint the areas where those two trigger points reside and give them hell. As with all of the other exercises the more consistent you are, the better results you will see.

The Triceps

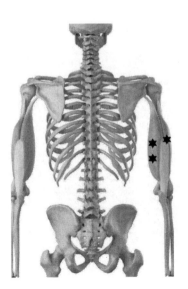

The triceps can be a seemingly insignificant source of shoulder pain, but I can assure you they have their part. As shown before, when the teres minor gets tight it will clamp down on the tricep tendon making it short and irritated. The shortness of the tricep muscle will now exert excessive pull on the back part of the shoulder. As a result people, will think their shoulder is the culprit. Remember, your shoulder pain is largely a symptom, not a problem. Treating the shoulder would be futile in the long run.

To do this mobilization you are going to once again start off on your back and place a softball under your tricep. There doesn't have to be too much rolling involved. Direct pressure tends to work the best.

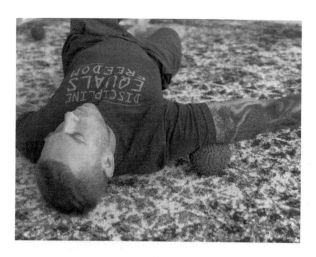

Place the ball in the areas I show where the trigger points develop. If they are in there, you will feel the pain start to travel into the shoulder or on down the arms. Trigger points in the tricep can be quite lively, so you shouldn't have to do too much searching. Spending 4-6 minutes at a time cleaning this area up should be plenty sufficient to get some relief. As with the other exercises, when you stop getting relief from the softball graduate to a baseball and then a lacrosse ball to completely diminish any tight, adhered tissue. Your shoulder will thank you for doing so!

Ask the Coach: What About Stretching the Shoulder?

One thing that you may have noticed and be scratching your head about is the fact that there is a lot of smashing of the muscles in this book but not a whole lot of stretching. Well, what gives? The reason why we do not stretch the muscles surrounding the shoulder is because the shoulder is a joint that relies heavily upon stability. Muscles are elastic, but the fascial sheet surrounding them is very plastic. While muscles will have the ability to retract due to their elastic nature, fascia does not.

When you introduce too much stretching to the shoulder joint, the muscles will become hypermobile. While that may sound like it's a good thing, people who are hypermobile get injured just as much as people who are tight. I work with four Yoga teachers on a regular basis for shoulder and wrist problems and surprise – they all teach around 3-5 classes per day.

There are two "stretching" mobilizations that I teach my clients in order to improve their range of motion and at the same time "reset" the muscles and tendons surrounding the joint. If you would like a video of me showing you how to do these two stretches please go to:
https://mailchi.mp/e2de0014017d/head-neck-shoulder
and enter your e-mail address in the box provided, and they will be sent right over to you pronto!

Chapter 4: Special Considerations

Anna came to me in shambles. Her constant headaches were keeping her from being able to focus at her high-stress job. Her shoulders were killing her, which was making it very difficult to do her work as well. It's no surprise that with these conditions she sat at a computer all day, but what was disheartening was that she told me she felt like she was starting to get depressed and her motivation was on the decline weekly.

Assessing Anna, I could not believe how tight her trap muscles were. It felt like they were both forged out of steel! Touching them lightly with the Back Buddy sent pain up into her head immediately surrounding her eye, and even referring some pain into her jaw. Anna talked about the eye strain to which I then asked her if she used any type of blue light blocking glasses. She had no idea what I was talking about.

I sent Anna away with specific instruction to buy a Back Buddy, gave her a set of exercises to do to break the tissue up surrounding her head and neck, and gave her a specific type of blue light blocking glasses to buy. Within three weeks, I followed up with her. As soon as she answered the phone I could tell she was already in a better space. She told me her headaches were down to nearly nothing and her shoulder pain was about 80 percent reduced. The inclusion of the blue light blocking glasses helped her retain significantly more energy through out her work day, and reduced her stress enough to where she actually had the vitality to start working out again. I wished her all the best and she was greatly appreciative for directing her to a higher level of health.

As the old saying goes – there is more than one way to skin a cat. I have found over the years that some issues that develop in the human body that practitioners love to label as "unfixable." Typically when people come to me with any type of pain - not just head, neck, and shoulder problems – I am able to successfully fix close to 95 percent of them. In cases like vertigo, motion sickness, or temporomandibular joint dysfunction, my success rate drops to around 75 percent.

In this section I am going to describe to you the exercises needed in order to drastically decrease the discomfort you are feeling with the afformentioned afflictions. Please be aware that we are working in very sensitive areas, on very sensitive conditions. I have had people come to me in tears with vertigo and TMJ dysfunction. Some of them I have been able to fix. Some of them got better and were happy with the limited results. Some of them I was not able to help and we called it after three sessions. If you are suffering from any of these afflictions, I hope you find some sort of relief or salvation in the methods that follow.

Motion Sickness

I suffered with motion sickness for many years when I was young. Whether it was the car, boat, or plane, they all made my head spin – literally. I can remember going on a boat and a plane in the same day and coming home to curl up on my grandmother's bed with the feeling that I am on a rocking boat. For some reason when I hit my teens the air sickness went away (I think it was because I actually visited a chiropractor and he adjusted my neck, which made my muscles less tense and my head straighter), but the seasickness never did get better. I would even get nauseated while surfing.

When I started to learn about how the muscles and nerves of the neck affect the head I started to do some experimenting, and to my surprise my scalenes were riddled with trigger points, and tight muscle tissue. As I started to work on my scalenes not only did my motion sickness start to get better, but my overall balance improved.

Here is my prescription for you if you have really bad motion sickness:

1. Work on your scalenes and your sternocleidomastoid. Your scalene muscles relate the position of your head in relation to your body back to your brain. If they are short on one side or have trigger points in

them, when you move your head your brain gets dizzy due to the unequal length on each side. Follow the mobility exercises for the scalenes, and SCM, and work on them as often as possible. Remember to be gentle and go slow. I recommend taking 3-5 days off from working on them periodically to give the brain a break from constantly having to recalibrate.
2. Work on the splenius muscles. When the muscles of the front of the neck get tight, the muscles in the back of the neck will tighten up as well so they don't lose the position of the head. Follow the mobility exercises for the splenius capitis and splenius cervicis. These can be maintained on a daily basis for a quick 4-5 minutes each time.
3. Work on the trapezius muscle. I find that when my traps get tight, I'll get nauseated even if I'm not on a moving vessel. Follow the mobility exercises I have listed for the traps to the best of your ability. You should really be mobilizing them every day, especially if you have a very stressful job, or if you are stressed out in general.
4. Work on fixing that atlas! When I fixed my atlas my motion sickness completely disappeared. I realize it's a very challenging task, but be diligent and do your best. If you run into any snags don't hesitate to contact me.

Vertigo

I have worked with three people who had vertigo. From what I gather, it is one of the worst feelings in the world. Vertigo can give someone the sensation that they are in a high, narrow staircase. They can become extremely dizzy, nauseated, and even vomit as a result. In every client who has come to see me complaining of this issue, I always find the same problem – ridiculously tight upper body muscles.

If you suffer from vertigo, here are the muscles you are going to want to focus on mobilizing to open up:

1. Scalenes & sternocleidomastoid
2. Splenius muscles
3. Trapezius muscles
4. Pectoralis minor & major
5. Levator scapulae
6. Rhomboids

In conjunction with doing those mobilizations, you may want to consider some naturally occuring supplement remedies as well. Two emerging supplements on today's market that help to deal with inflammation and stress are CBD oil, and curcumin. The best type of CBD oil I have found is made by Charlotte's Web and you can find it at http://www.cwhemp.com. It is made specifically from hemp and does not contain the psychotropic substance THC that Cannabis does, so you can rest assured you will not test positive for any illegal substances. Tim Ferriss even plugged this supplement for helping cure a three-day insomnia bender he was not too excited to be going through.

    I heard about clinical trials of curcumin blowing the socks off of the scientists that were studying it more than four years ago. Curcumin is found in the root turmeric, but you would need to eat close to five pounds of it per day to get the desired amount two capsules will give you. It is also the compound that turns curry dishes yellow. Curcumin is being found to create the following benefits to the human body:

1. Decrease inflammation.
2. Decrease risk of heart attack.
3. Increases brain-derived neurotrophic factor, which increases brain function.
4. Increase the antioxidant capacity of the body.
5. Can help prevent and maybe help treat cancer.
6. Prevent and treat Alzheimer's disease.
7. Help decrease the symptoms of arthritis.
8. Helps decrease the incidence of depression by controlling inflammation.
9. May help delay the aging process.
10. Has many other medicinal properties.

I had surgery on my left knee in 2015 when a weightlifting accident occurred. I took 1500mgs of curcumin for three weeks leading up to the surgery, then uped it to 3000 mgs after the surgery. When I went back to the doctor three days after surgery to get my dressing off and stitches out ,the nurse was amazed at the lack of inflammation in my knee. After seeing that, I was sold on curcumin and take it every day now. You can get the brand of curcumin I personally use from the Chris approved supplement section on my website www.chriskidawski.com

TMJ

Temporomandibular joint dysfunction can range from a slight click to a major crunch/pop when the mouth opens and closes. While the mechanisms dealing with this dysfunction are beyond the scope of this book, there are some easy maneuvers you can do in order to alleviate or even get rid of that annoying little click in your jaw.

Mobilize your Temporalis

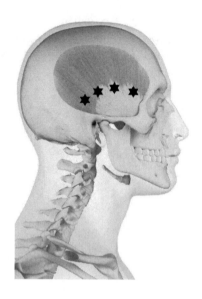

As you can see by that nice little rainbow of trigger points, the temporalis muscle be a huge factor when it comes to headaches, but what about jaw pain or TMJ? Well the easiest way to find out is to put your finger on your temporalis and then open and close your mouth. Can you feel the tissue slide under your finger? When the temporalis develops trigger points or tightness it will pull on the muscles of the jaw causing them to be shorter as well.

To mobilize this area, you are going to need two lacrosse balls. I want you to lay down on your side and support your head with the lacrosse ball on your temporalis. You are then going to take the other lacrosse ball and place it on the temporalis on the other side and then open and close your mouth for a minute or two.

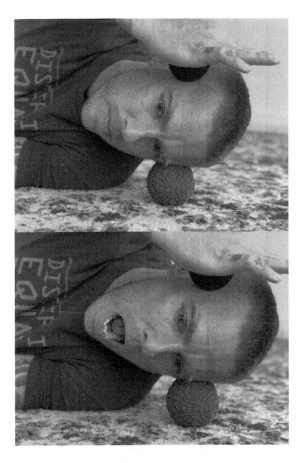

Be aware this may make your jaw click a little louder, and it may even be painful. This is because you are shortening up the muscle even more. By continuously doing this exercise you will slowly start to open the trigger points up and lengthen the muscle. Once this is accomplished, we can now work on the actual jaw itself.

The Lateral Pterygoid

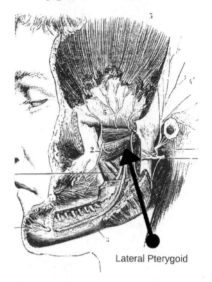

Lateral Pterygoid

    The lateral pterygoid is such an under appreciated muscle that this was the only medically accurate photo I could find on my royalty free picture website. If it is a little bit challenging to read that's ok because it's from 1885! The lateral pterygoid is obviously a major muscle involved in chewing, and it would therefore be even more obvious that if it starts to get tight or dysfunction, we will get a nice little click in the jaw or develop TMJ.

    When TMJ dysfunction occurs we have a space problem. The lower jawbone essentially gets sucked up and in creating grinding, popping and cracking. In order to help loosen this up you are going to press your knuckles into both sides of your jaw and pull down on the tissue.

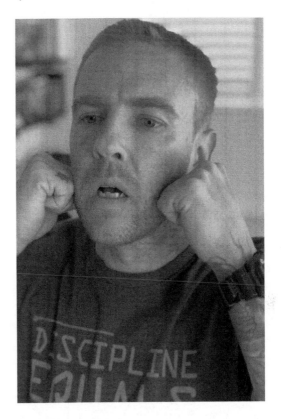

Work the tissue in a downward motion for 3-5 minutes depending on how sore and tender everything is. You can do this 3-5 times per day as well; the more you get the tissue surrounding the jaw to relax the better.

The Masseter

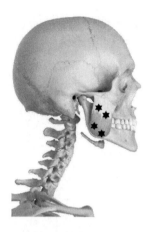

You would think that you would be able to mobilize the masseter in the same manner as the lateral pterygoid just by looking at where it is oriented, and you would be partly right. The two trigger points located at the bottom of the muscle can be easily grinded into with your knuckles. The two trigger points at the top however require a little more finesse.

To start off you are going to want to wash your hands thoroughly because in order to mobilize the affected area of your masseter you are going to have to stick your finger in your mouth. Using your thumb and index finger you are then going to pinch and massage the masseter muscle from the inside and outside of your mouth.

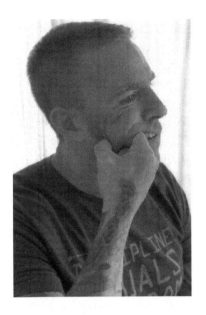

Play around with the tissue and see if one side feels different than the other. Work this mobilization for 3-5 minutes, concentrating on any tender areas and try to get as much movement out of the jaw as you can.

Concluding Thoughts

These days, stress can be a person's number-one enemy. As intangible as it is, stress does a very good job at making some things appear real when they are not, or amplifying other things when they are small. Oftentimes this worry manifests itself as head, neck, and shoulder pain as our body unconsciously collapses in an effort to become as small as possible to deal with seemingly insurmountable issues. Growing up in the American way, I understand the habit of being hard on yourself and sometimes on your loved ones as well. When we are experiencing pain on a daily basis as a result of this stress, sometimes we don't want to incur more pain to get rid of. With that in mind, here are a couple of recommendations to help de-pressurize your life more gently.

1. Visit a float tank – Float tanks provide you with a sensation – less atmosphere. It is 100% soundproof, and the water is mixed with magnesium to make you feel weightless at a steady 98.6 degrees. There is no light in the tank either. When these senses have nothing to do your ability to listen to your body will be amplified. Feel your tight areas and decipher where your pain is coming from. Relax and meditate on something constructive/positive.
2. Sit in a sauna/hot tub/infrared sauna – The benefits of any type of sauna are amazing. You will increase your circulation/heart rate, and sweat out toxins not to mention heat your muscles up and make them more pliable. While I do not recommend mobilizing in a sauna – feel free to do so, but other people may look at you strange. I always use strange stares as an opportunity to teach!
3. Take a meditation vacation – The best decision I have ever made in my life was to take a meditation vacation. I stayed in a

beautiful house just outside of the town of Assisi in Italy. We meditated twice per day, guided by a lovely husband and wife. I came back to the states a newly revived man thanks to that vacation and have continued my meditation practice to this day.

4. Walk in the park or beach barefoot – A large part of our pain can come from losing our connection with the Earth. The Earth contains a high concentration of negative ions, which when absorbed by the body create a healing effect unlike that of any medicine on the planet. To absorb these ions we must be barefoot on grass, soil, sand, or immersed in a lake, pond, or the sea. The problem is most of us never let our feet touch the actual ground due to our footwear, or living in a high rise building. I try to spend 15-30 minutes grounded every day while walking or playing with my dog. There are also many grounding sheets you can purchase on the Internet for your bed.

5. Take a quality Vitamin D3 supplement – Research studies show that soft tissue injuries are more likely to occur in people who have low Vitamin D levels. Vitamin D is actually a hormone that is responsible for over 90 genetic processes in your body. If you are not spending a large amount of time in the sun, then I highly recommend you start to supplement as soon as possible. You can

buy the brand I personally use by going to my website.

Your head, neck, or shoulder pain does not have to be a death sentence. Making it through this book has given you more information than 99 percent of the population has. Be consistent in employing the methods and don't give up. If you are experiencing a very challenging situation I have not addressed in this book, please to set up a free consultation with me on my website under the pain management tab.

With gratitude to your health,

CK
Owner/CEO
Influential Health Solutions

About The Author

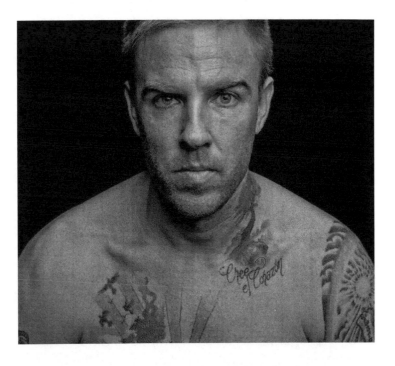

Chris Kidawski has been transforming lives in the health and fitness profession for the last 20 years. Armed with his master's in Kinesiology from the University of Hawai'i he helps heal and reverse disease from the inside out. Chris has trained people in all walks of life including but not limited to Navy SEALs, professional athletes, World Champion mixed martial artists, mothers, fathers, sons, daughters, and people just like you!

Chris has dedicated himself to discovering the truth about all aspects of health and wellness and has become as complete of a life coach as you can get. He has written many books on the topic of health and wellness - most notably The Death Of Dieting, which teaches you how to lose weight and detoxify your body with natural, wholesome food, The Everspace, which teaches you how to operate from a place of stillness to achieve success in your life, and The Back Pain Bible, which is a breakthrough step by step process to eradicate chronic lower back pain. All are sitting on Amazon best-seller lists!

Chris now lives and runs his business Influential Health Solutions from sunny South Florida, but also does public speaking engagements and seminars in Universities, Corporations, and gyms all over the country. He has been featured on many podcasts where he dives deeper into his body/spirit/mind paradigm of human health and thoroughly enjoys opening up people's lives with his information. For speaking engagements contact Chris at rebuildingu@proton.me

Printed in Poland
by Amazon Fulfillment
Poland Sp. z o.o., Wrocław

29574019R00067